DASH Diet Essentials

Hanna Davis

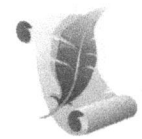

DASH Diet Essentials

A Beginner's Guide to the DASH Diet with a Proven Lifestyle Plan and Delicious Recipes so You Can Lower Your Blood Pressure, Lose Weight, Feel Great and Live a Healthy Life

Softpress Publishing

SOFTPRESS PUBLISHING
4118 Hickory Crossroads Road
Kenly, NC 27542
softpresspub@gmail.com

ISBN-13: 978-1-5002-8589-0
ISBN-10: 1-5002-8589-7

Disclaimer:
This product is not intended to diagnose, treat, cure, or prevent any disease. The advice and strategies contained herein may not be suitable for every situation. This work is sold with the understanding that the publisher is not engaged in rendering medical or other professional advice or services. The publisher does not specifically endorse any company or product mentioned or cited in this document. Websites listed were accurate at the time of publishing but may have changed or disappeared between when it was written and when it is read.

No responsibility or liability is assumed by the publisher for any injury, damage or financial loss sustained to persons or property from the use of this information, personal or otherwise, either directly or indirectly. While every effort has been made to ensure reliability and accuracy of the information within, all liability, negligence or otherwise, from any use, misuse or abuse of the operation of any methods, strategies, instructions or ideas contained in the material herein, is sole responsibility of the reader.

All information is generalized, presented for informational purposes only and presented "as is" without warranty or guarantee of any kind.

All trademarks and brands referred to in this book are for illustrative purposes only, are the property of their respective owners and not affiliated with this publication in any way.

Table of Contents

Introduction

Before you roll your eyes and think, "Not another fad diet," you need to read this. This is not a fad diet. There are no empty promises that you will look like Cindy Crawford or Jason Statham in just a matter of weeks after you adopt the diet. You are not going to lose 100 pounds in a month or even three months. No, the DASH diet isn't about that. It is all about making you healthier, which in turn will result in some weight loss. Consider it a healthy lifestyle change more than a diet. Your body will thank you.

DASH stands for—Dietary Approaches to Stop Hypertension.

It was developed based on research gleaned from the National Heart, Lung and Blood Institute's studies. The diet is designed to lower high blood pressure without the use of medicines. A proper diet can do that while increasing healthy fats in the bloodstream. This is important to reducing the risk of heart disease.

The diet does not involve you living off lemonade or drinking juice for seven days straight. There are no crazy tricks or extreme restrictions to make this diet work. You can still eat most of the foods you love. You don't have to feel as if cardboard-tasting food is your only option.

So, let's dive right in and learn more about this new lifestyle plan you are going to undertake.

One last thing, as a way of saying Thank You for buying my book, I have put together a **free** gift just for you!

"23 DASH Diet Snacks"

This gift is the perfect complement to this book, so just head over to this web address to get the free download:

https://tinyurl.com/35parn58

Chapter 1

What is the DASH Diet?

The DASH diet operates on the principle that food is good for your body. It is simply cutting back on foods that are high in sodium. The only serious restriction of the diet is making sure you don't eat more than 2,300 grams of sodium in a single day. Keeping that in mind, folks who already have high blood pressure, are over 51 years of age, have kidney disease or diabetes will want to lower that number to 1,500 grams of sodium. African Americans are at higher risk of high blood pressure and should also aim for a daily sodium intake of 1,500 grams. It is important to mention that these limits are based on a daily calorie intake of 2,000. Higher or lower caloric intakes will need some adjusting, and we will address that later in the book.

The diet clearly works and has managed to receive the "#1 Diet" by the US News & Report for four years in a row. It has gained this prestigious placement at the top because it is all about making you healthy first and worrying about your thunder thighs second. In case you are still not convinced the diet is good for you and works, the American Heart Association also recommends it.

The DASH diet isn't only for your parents or the groups mentioned above. Children, athletes, and healthy people alike can all benefit from restricting their sodium intake and eating a diet rich in fresh fruits and vegetables. The idea is to give your body everything it needs to stay in tip top shape. Magnesium, potassium and calcium are all necessary for a healthy body and can lower blood pressure naturally. Fruits and veggies are packed with these healthy nutrients and let's be honest, munching on strawberries is a lot more fun than popping vitamins.

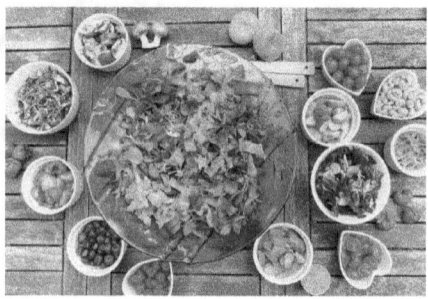

Benefits of the DASH Diet

That is kind of a given—better health! You knew that, but you want specifics. We have already covered one of the major benefits to the diet, but there is so much more. There is a bit of a trickle effect when you choose to lower your sodium intake to a level that is healthy. When you think of your grandparents, your parents or even yourself if you are over the age of 40, you probably have some concerns about blood pressure levels. In our society, that is normal. We are told we need to monitor our blood pressure after a certain age. It is actually very normal to be at a dinner or other social gathering and actually discuss the topic of one's blood pressure.

*Having high blood pressure puts you at risk of heart attack and stroke. By ensuring your blood pressure is at a healthy level, you can reduce the chances of suffering either one of those. By following the DASH diet, your systolic number (the bottom number on your blood pressure) can drop anywhere from 7 to 12 points. This is a huge benefit to your overall health.

*Another benefit is a healthy diet will reduce your risk of diabetes. One of the major contributors to diabetes is an unhealthy diet that throws the body out of whack. The body doesn't use the insulin produced, and you suffer a number of nasty side effects, including diabetes.

*Osteoporosis is another one of those diseases we almost expect to face in old age. You don't have to if you keep your body in tip top shape. Eating a low-sodium diet can do that.

*Cancer is another horrific disease that seems to be on the rise plaguing all those we love. We are warned against smoking, drinking and a whole long list of things that increase our risk of cancer. A healthy diet is one way to reduce the risk of developing certain cancers including colorectal and estrogen receptor negative breast cancer in women. The DASH diet is an effective tool in the fight against cancer.

*You will lose weight on the DASH diet, but that is not what it was designed for. A healthy weight is part of being in good shape which translates to a reduced risk of the above-mentioned illnesses.

*The risk of developing painful kidney stones is dropped nearly in half for men and women who follow the DASH diet. The diet also slows down the progression of early stage kidney disease.

These conditions interrupt your life and can ultimately cut it short. Taking the time to learn how to feed your body properly is essential to living out a full, complete life.

Chapter 2

Basics of the DASH Diet

At first glance, the DASH diet can seem a little intimidating. You can get very technical with your diet and monitor every calorie and where it comes from. In fact, in the beginning, you will want to keep a food diary to help you learn more about what you eat on a normal basis. Understanding where your calories come from will help you figure out what you need to cut out from your regular diet and where to supplement.

The following is a chart that helps explain how the DASH diet is configured. Don't panic and automatically assume it is far too complicated for you to follow. You don't need to carry a calculator around with you, but you do need to be conscience of what you are eating. There is a learning curve, but once you get the hang of it, it will become second nature to you.

Total fat	27% of calories
Saturated fat	6% of calories
Protein	18% of calories
Carbohydrate	55% of calories
Cholesterol	150 mg
Sodium	2,300 mg
Potassium	4,700 mg
Calcium	1,250 mg
Magnesium	500 mg
Fiber	30 g

BASICS OF THE DASH DIET

Another way to look at the diet is as follows:

Grains - 4 to 6 servings a day
Vegetables - 4 to 5 servings a day
Fruits - 4 to 5 servings a day
Dairy - 2 to 3 servings a day
Lean meat, fish and poultry - Kept under 6 servings a day
Nuts, seeds and beans - 4 to 5 servings a week
Sweets - Less than 5 a week
Oils and fats - 2 to 3 servings a day

The idea is to lower blood pressure to a safe level without relying on prescription medications to do so. By eating a diet rich in foods that do this naturally, you are effectively taking care of several problems at once. Your blood pressure will drop, your cholesterol levels will drop, and you will drop some weight. These three things are crucial to your overall health. And, getting these things in line can reduce your risk of other, more serious health problems. Doesn't it sound more appealing to eat more fruits and vegetable than taking pills every day that make you feel sick and tired?

Part of the problem in today's world is we opt for foods that are quick and easy without real concern for the actual nutritional value. We are missing out on some valuable nutrients that our bodies need to thrive. Overtime, the lack in nutrients causes serious problems that manifest in a variety of diseases and conditions. The DASH diet isn't only about reducing blood pressure. It also addresses the lack of vitamins and minerals in the daily diet. By removing processed foods and replacing them with fresh fruits and vegetables and lean meats, we are giving our bodies what it needs to operate in tip-top shape.

To help tailor the DASH diet to you and your lifestyle, you need to ask yourself a couple of questions.

1-What is your activity level on a daily basis?

Sedentary lifestyles would mean you are relatively inactive the majority of the day.

Moderately active means you do some light activity and walk the equivalent of a mile to 3 miles a day.

Active means you do activity that is equal to walking more than 3 miles a day on top of your regular light duty activities.

Once you have chosen your activity level, you can figure out how much food you need on a given day to keep up with your lifestyle. As is typical for any diet, men and women will have different calorie needs.

Gender	Calories Needed for Each Activity Level			
	Age (years)	Sedentary	Moderately Active	Active
Female	19–30	2,000	2,000–2,200	2,400
	31–50	1,800	2,000	2,200
	51+	1,600	1,800	2,000–2,200
Male	19–30	2,400	2,600–2,800	3,000
	31–50	2,200	2,400–2,600	2,800–3,000
	51+	2,000	2,200–2,400	2,400–2,800

Credit: http://www.nhlbi.nih.gov/health/public/heart/hbp/dash/dash_brief.htm

2-What do I normally eat on a given day?

To understand this, you will want to keep a food journal for a minimum of 3 days. Track what you eat and drink each day. It is simple and helpful if you use one of the free calorie counting programs or apps available on iTunes or the Google Playstore. The programs will figure out all the details and make it easy to track.

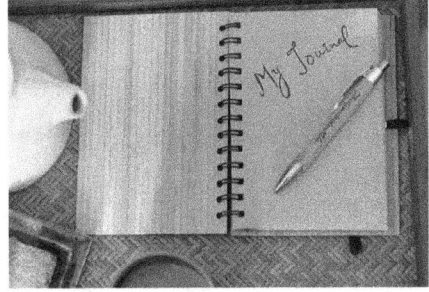

After tracking your typical diet for a few days, you will need to go back and evaluate it to determine where you need to cut back. Remember, it isn't only about calories. It is the type of calories that you are consuming that truly matter. Refer to the chart on page 4 to understand this a little better. With one of those handy calorie trackers, you won't have to worry about doing any of the calculating. It will all be done for you.

Please don't get too hung up on the numbers. That can seem overwhelming and may deter you from the diet. The charts are a guideline. Later in the book you will find recipes that you can incorporate into your meal plan that will help you stay within the DASH diet guidelines. It is all about changing the way you eat, just as you would institute a new healthy habit or eliminate an unhealthy one. It will take some practice, but soon you will be eating healthy without putting a lot of thought into it.

Chapter 3

Foods to Avoid

A diet wouldn't really be a diet if you could just eat and drink everything you pleased without worrying about the negative consequences. Fortunately, the DASH diet isn't so hung up on counting calories that you miss out on some of your favorite foods. I'm sure you've heard before, it's all about moderation. You can eat a wide variety of foods, including some of your favorite treats, as long as you don't sit down with a tub of ice cream and a spoon and go to town.

With that said, there are some foods you will want to avoid in order to stay in line with the DASH diet guidelines. Don't panic! The list is not too long, and you will find plenty of substitutes to take the place of the foods you are missing.

Sugars

Sugar is a big no-no on any diet. It isn't good for you, and it is fattening. You may not even realize some of the food you eat on a regular basis is loaded with refined sugar. You are going to need to start paying attention to labels. Some common foods that are high in sugar include: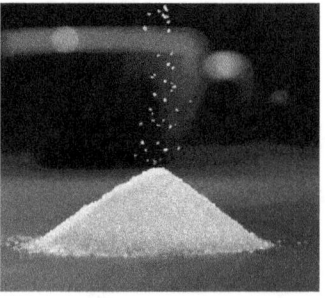

- Pastries, cookies, cakes – basically anything made with white flour and processed;

- Soda and some fruit juices;

- Syrup—maple, agave, molasses;

- Candy;

- White breads and rolls are often high in sugar—read the labels.

Fats

Fatty foods are another diet no-brainer. However, there are some fats that are good for you, like the Omega-3s, but others, like the following, that should be limited:

- Trans-fats are typically found in ready-to-eat foods including crackers and sweet snacks;

- Saturated fats are not visible, you will need to read labels. Avoid coconut and palm oil;

- Omega-6 oils include vegetable oil, safflower oil, corn and soybean oil;

- Butter should be very limited.

Caffeine

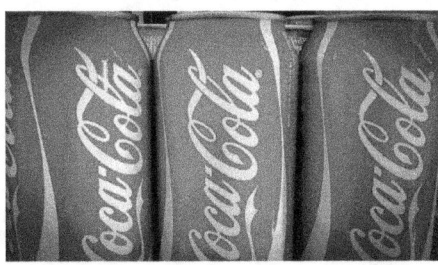 Caffeine will dehydrate the body and should be avoided as much as possible. Sodas, teas and coffees are often rich in caffeine. Check the labels and opt for decaffeinated and sugar-free beverages, or avoid the following altogether:

- Coffee;

- Energy drinks;

- Tea;

- Chocolate;

- Chocolate or coffee-flavored ice cream.

Salt

The DASH diet focuses on low sodium so that means you are going to need to cut out foods high in sodium. Beware of salt substitutes that are high in potassium. The idea is to reduce your salt intake to a healthy level without overdoing the amount of potassium you digest which can cause other health problems. These foods are typically high in salt content:

- Potato chips;

- Soy sauce;

- Canned meats;

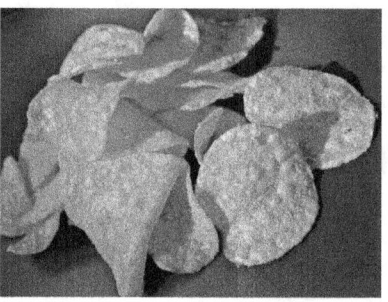

- Frozen meals i.e. burritos and pizza;

- Salted nuts;

- Canned foods like ravioli, spaghetti and chili;

- Canned beans and other vegetables.

This is a rather short list when you think about the amount of food that is currently available to us. Don't get hung up on what you shouldn't eat. Instead, focus on all the great things you can eat without hurting your body and damaging your health.

Chapter 4

Planning Your DASH Diet Transition

Any transition is going to have some really awesome perks and a few drawbacks. Fortunately, your transition to a healthier way of eating is mostly going to be smooth, and you will soon start to feel the difference in your daily routines. You will have more energy. You will look and feel better, and your overall quality of life will increase. But, it would be neglectful not to point out that as you transition your diet from one laden with starchy, sugary carbohydrates to one filled with fresh fruits and vegetables, you are going to experience 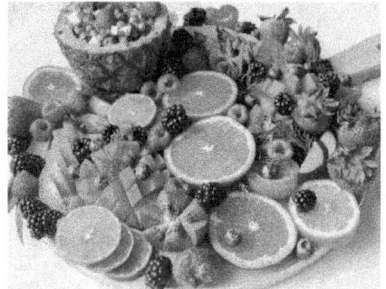 something you may not totally appreciate.

Fresh fruits and veggies are rich in natural fiber. That means there are going to be some digestive changes. Don't worry, the extra trips to the bathroom are short-lived. Your body will need to adjust to the healthier lifestyle and will need to get rid of some of the stuff that has been bogging down your digestive system. This phase will likely last a week or two. Don't give up because the benefits of eating a healthy diet far outweigh this one minor, short-lived inconvenience.

Slowly Change Your Diet

The first week will be more about reducing your sodium intake while increasing the amount of fresh fruit and vegetables. In the next chapter, you will learn some tips about how to do that without completely altering your regular diet.

The transition will also include phasing out that loaf of white bread in the pantry. When it is gone, buy a loaf of whole grain bread to replace it. The slow transition will help lessen some of the side effects of switching to a high fiber diet.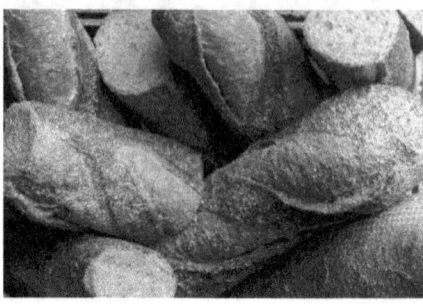

During this transitional period, you may also want to invest in some anti-bloating and gas over-the-counter medicines to make it a little more tolerable. Don't get scared and reject the diet! This is just part of cleaning out your system and getting rid of all the nasty stuff that is making you unhealthy.

Goal-Setting and Rewards

In order to be successful with sticking to the DASH diet, you need to set goals and rewards. The goals you set depend on what you want to achieve but should be realistic and measurable. An example might be to lose 2 pounds in the first 2 weeks on the diet. Or, you may establish an exercise goal of walking 1 mile each day in your first week. Then, increase it from there as you begin to make progress.

Each time you reach a goal, you should reward yourself. This will give you something to look forward to as you strive for reaching your goals. One of your rewards could be a small shopping spree. You are going to need a new wardrobe to compliment your shrinking figure. Another reward option could be something much cheaper, like a trip to the movies, or a round of golf on that course you have been dreaming about.

Whatever you decide, your goals should challenge you, and your rewards should motivate you. This is because the first few weeks of your transition from an unhealthy way of eating to the DASH diet will be the most challenging. And, rewarding yourself when you reach a goal will keep you on track.

The good news is that you will lose a few pounds, and there is a real possibility you will drop a size or two! However, don't beat yourself up for slipping up. You are human, and mistakes are part of life. The diet isn't meant to punish you by leaving you feeling hungry and deprived. There will be times when you indulge, but don't scrap the diet because you think you have just blown it. You haven't! Always look forward!

Exercise

Add in exercise as part of the transitional process. Although the main goal isn't to lose weight, your body needs regular activity to stay in top condition. Change your existing routine to incorporate 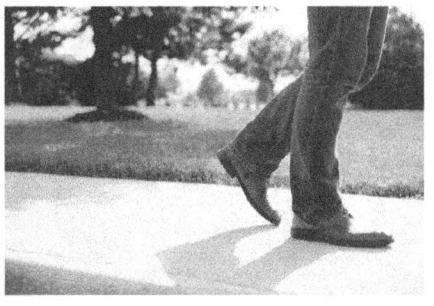 a little more physical activity. You don't have to buy a gym membership or run on the treadmill for an hour a day. Little things like taking a walk after dinner instead of sitting down and watching television for a couple of hours is helpful.

Take the stairs instead of the elevator at work. Park your car farther out in the parking lot at the grocery store or mall so you can get some extra walking in. Walk to the corner market to pick up that gallon of milk instead of driving. The goal is to get at least 30 minutes of exercise a day. If you don't have the time or the ability to get all your exercise requirements in one block, break it up into ten-minute blocks. You will need to make a conscience effort to do this.

All of these things are great for your health and you will start to feel good about the choices you are making to be healthier. If you have children, you are teaching them how to live healthy, and they will hopefully be able to avoid some of the problems many of our parents and grandparents deal with.

Chapter 5

Tips to Upholding the DASH Diet

Okay, now let's talk about how you can maintain your DASH diet goal. If you don't have a personal chef who has been trained on how to cook delicious meals that meet the diet requirements, you are going to need to learn how to cook your own healthy meals. You are also going to need to know what to buy to make your meals a little healthier. And for those occasions when you go out for a meal, you need to know what your options are. You are not going to be regulated to a plain Caesar salad while those around you chow down on steaks and buttery potatoes and rolls.

Cooking

There is one mistake many people make when they try a new diet. They think their tastes are going to change. They won't. If you don't like broccoli today, you are not going to like it tomorrow. You need to choose recipes that appeal to you and your particular tastes. Look for substitutes with similar vegetables and meats that will make the recipe work for you. If you don't like spinach, try kale and things like that. With that said, the following tips will help you choose the right recipes to keep you happy on your DASH diet.

- Keep your favorite recipes but tweak them to make them a little healthier. Use low-fat and low-sodium ingredients and fresh foods rather than canned or processed foods.

- Use healthier meat cuts or skip the meat altogether. This is easy to do with pasta dishes like spaghetti and lasagna.

- Don't automatically salt your dishes before you even try them. If a recipe calls for a ½ teaspoon of salt, omit it. Chances are you won't even taste the difference.

- Experiment with herbs for seasoning. You would be amazed at the difference fresh herbs and spices can make to a dish. They are so flavorful you won't need salt at all.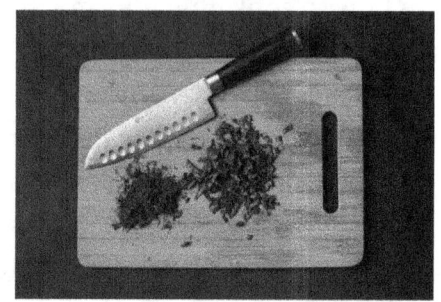

- Use nonstick cookware to limit the need for cooking oils, sprays and butter.

- Invest in a steamer and grill to cook healthier. Steamed vegetables retain more nutrients than boiled and are healthier than sautéed or fried veggies. Grills are the ideal way to cook fish, chicken and lean cuts of meat.

- Rinse off vegetables that have been in a can. This will help wash away some of the excess salt that is used in the canning process.

Shopping

When you head out to the supermarket, you are going to need to change up your routine a bit. It is easy to get into a rut when you go shopping. You grab your cart and head for the produce section, before picking up your meats and then your breads or something like that. You probably don't even really think much about what you toss in your cart. It is typically the same stuff every week. But no more!

Now, you are heading into your grocery store with a fresh set of eyes and a new mission—to eat healthy! You don't need to do the up and down method of shopping. In fact, the majority of your time will be spent in the perimeter of your grocery store. Dairy, meat and produce will make up the bulk of your cart. Make a list and stick to it. Review all the recipes you are going to be using and don't deviate from the ingredient list.

- Buy more produce than usual. In fact, make it about a third of your total groceries for the week. Instead of one bunch of bananas, buy two. Buy 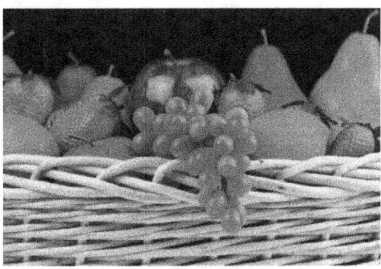 apples, oranges, carrots and other fresh fruits and veggies you like. Try some new ones as well.

- Buy less meat. Meat isn't going to be the focus of your meals any longer. Your meals are going to include a variety of fruits, veggies, whole grains and meat. Your goal is less than 6 ounces of meat a day (think about the size of a deck of playing cards). Lean meats, chicken and fresh fish are all good choices. Choose skinless chicken when possible to make life a little easier.

- Skip the canned soups. They are high in sodium. If you must, choose low-sodium or no sodium options. Buy the ingredients necessary to make your own soups. It is rather easy to do.

- Don't even bother walking down the junk food aisle. There is nothing you need there. If you really need a quick, salty snack, head to the health food or natural food section and grab some rice cakes or rice snaps that will satisfy that craving.

- Choose cooking oils that are low in sodium. Your best bet is extra virgin olive oil.

- In the dairy section, choose low-fat or fat-free products like sour cream and cream cheese. Low-fat milk and yogurt are widely available as well. Organic is also a great choice.

- In the pasta section, choose whole-grain varieties. Whole-grain rice is also a better option over the quick minute-rice varieties.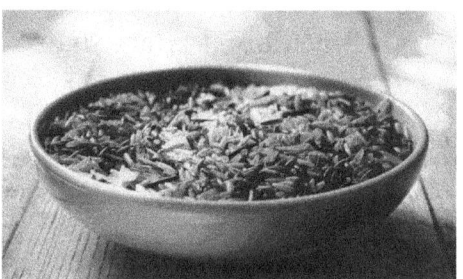

Dining Out

Eating out can be a bit of a chore when you are on a strict diet. Fortunately, the DASH diet is not overly strict, and you can still enjoy a meal prepared by somebody else while enjoying the company of friends and family. Many restaurants now feature menu items that include calorie count as well as sodium numbers. This makes it easy for you to pick and choose meals that are in line with the DASH program.

- Opt for water with your meal or a club soda. With this one decision you are limiting your salt intake.

- Order an appetizer that focuses on fresh fruits and vegetables rather than anything deep fried.

- For your salad course, ask for the dressing to be placed on the side. Ask that there not be any cheese, meats or eggs. A spinach salad or some simple greens are actually rather tasty.

- Breads are often offered in whole grain varieties. If that is not an option and you really want a roll or breadstick, go for it, but eat it dry without butter. Stick to just one and you will be okay.

- Choose a main dish with meat that is grilled, baked or broiled (but not in butter). Ask for steamed vegetables as a side dish 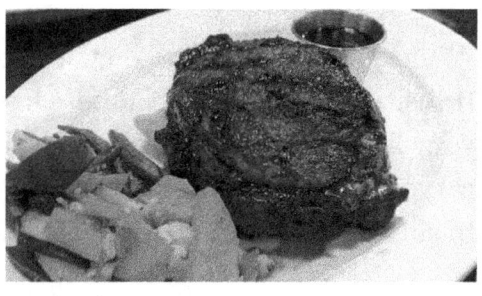 instead of white rice or mashed potatoes with butter. If baked potatoes are available, that is an option, but you will need to go easy on the butter and salt.

As you can see, these are not major life changes you need to make. It is simply thinking twice before ordering a meal or heading to the grocery store. You can still enjoy delicious food without all the extra stuff that you have become accustomed to. Your palate will adjust to your decision to limit the salt. Food may taste a little bland at first, but in a matter of weeks you won't even notice. It is all about changing your mindset. You can program your brain to like food without a bunch of salt, pepper and butter. It is refreshing to eat food as it was intended instead of doctored beyond recognition.

Chapter 6

Recipes

This chapter is packed with an assortment of recipes that you are sure to love. You won't find recipes that require 4 years of culinary school to make nor will you find recipes with ingredients you would have to search high and low for.

When going on a new diet, the key is to make it a smooth transition that is easy to adhere to without completely changing your life. The recipes are arranged by meal times of day so you can put together your own weekly meal plans. That is essential to staying within the DASH diet parameters.

Plan out your meals for a whole week. Make a shopping list to collect all the ingredients you will need. You will probably have to look twice at these "healthy" recipes. They resemble the food you eat today, with a few modifications to make them healthier, but just as delicious.

Breakfast

Baked Spiced Apple Oatmeal

Ingredients

    1 egg, beaten
    ½ cup applesauce
    1½ cups non-fat or 1% milk
    1 teaspoon vanilla
    2 tablespoons oil
    1 apple, chopped
    2 cups rolled oats

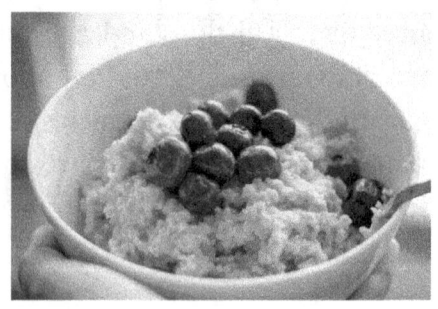

1 teaspoon baking powder

¼ teaspoon salt

1 teaspoon cinnamon

Optional topping

2 tablespoons brown sugar

2 tablespoons chopped nuts

Blueberries or raspberries

Directions:

1. Preheat oven to 375 degrees.
2. Prepare an 8x8 inch baking pan by spraying with a low-fat cooking spray.
3. Mix egg, applesauce, milk, vanilla and oil in a small mixing bowl. Stir in apple chunks.
4. In a small bowl, combine oats, baking powder, salt and cinnamon.
5. Add dry ingredients to applesauce mixture.
6. Add mixture to the baking dish and bake for 25 minutes.
7. Remove from oven and add toppings if desired. Return to oven to broil for 3 minutes until toppings are crunchy.

Bread Pudding-Breakfast Style

Ingredients

1½ cup low fat 1% or fat free milk

4 eggs

2 tablespoons brown sugar

½ teaspoon vanilla extract

½ teaspoon ground cinnamon

$1/_8$ teaspoon salt

3 cups cubed whole wheat bread, about 4 slices

½ cup peeled and diced apple

¼ cup raisins

Directions:

1. Preheat oven to 350 degrees.
2. Prepare 8x8 inch baking pan by spraying with cooking spray.
3. Combine milk, eggs, sugar, vanilla, cinnamon and salt in a large bowl. Stir well.
4. Add in the bread, apple and raisins and mix again. Bread should be coated with wet ingredients.
5. Pour mixture into prepared pan and cover with foil.
6. Cook for 40 minutes.
7. Remove the foil and continue baking for another 20 minutes.

On-the-Go Peanut Butter Smoothie

Ingredients

1 cup nonfat milk

1 tablespoon peanut butter

1 medium banana, frozen or fresh

Directions:

1. Place all ingredients in a blender and mix until smooth.
2. Pour it in your favorite to-go cup, and you have a healthy breakfast on the go.

Breakfast Fruit Salad

Ingredients

3 cups water

¾ cup quick cooking brown rice

¾ cup bulgur

1 Granny Smith apple

1 Red Delicious apple

1 orange

1 cup raisins

1 container (8-ounce) low-fat vanilla yogurt

Directions:

1. Bring water to a boil in a large pot.
2. Add rice and bulgur; Reduce to a simmer and cook for 10 minutes.
3. Remove from heat and let rest for 2 minutes.
4. Spread rice mixture onto a cooking sheet and allow to cool completely.
5. Chop apples and peel the orange before cutting into slices.
6. Dump the grains into a bowl and add fruit and yogurt. Mix well and serve.

Banana Pancakes

<u>Ingredients</u>

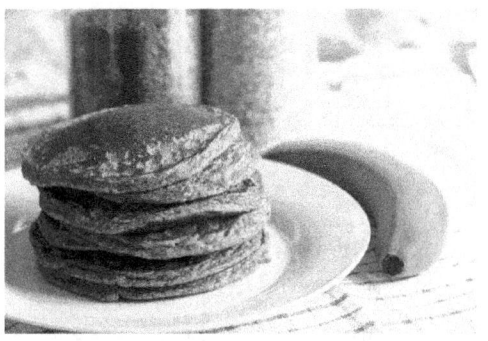

1 cup whole wheat flour

2 tsp baking powder

¼ tsp salt

¼ tsp cinnamon

1 large banana, mashed

1 cup 1% milk

3 large egg whites

2 tsp oil

1 tsp vanilla

2 tbsp chopped walnuts

<u>Directions:</u>

1. Mix flour, baking powder, salt and cinnamon in a large bowl.
2. In a separate bowl, mix milk, egg whites, oil, vanilla and mashed banana until smooth.
3. Pour into dry ingredients and mix well. Add in chopped nuts.
4. Pour ¼ cup of batter onto a griddle and cook approximately 3 minutes on each side or until done.
5. Try topping your pancakes with fresh fruit or yogurt instead of syrup.

Green Breakfast Smoothie

Ingredients

- 1 medium banana
- 1 cup baby spinach, packed
- ½ cup fat-free milk
- ¼ cup whole oats
- ¾ cup frozen mango
- ¼ cup plain nonfat yogurt
- ½ teaspoon vanilla

Directions:

Mix all ingredients in a blender and blend until smooth.

French Toast with Applesauce

Ingredients

- 4 egg whites
- ½ cup milk
- 1 teaspoon ground cinnamon
- 2 tablespoons white sugar
- ¼ cup unsweetened applesauce
- 6 slices whole wheat bread

Directions:

1. Mix egg whites, milk, cinnamon, sugar and applesauce in a bowl.
2. Dip bread slices in mixture one at a time until coated.
3. Spray griddle with a nonstick cooking spray.
4. Cook bread on each side for approximately 3 minutes or until golden brown.
5. Top with fresh fruit or a spoonful of applesauce, if desired. Blueberries or strawberries are a great choice.

Turkey Sausage Frittata
(make ahead recipe)

Ingredients

8 ounces wheat bread, cut into 1-inch cubes

12 ounces turkey sausage

2 cups fat free milk

1½ cup (4 ounces) reduced-fat shredded sharp cheddar cheese

3 large eggs

12 ounces egg substitute

½ cup chopped green onion

1 cup sliced mushrooms

½ teaspoon paprika

Fresh ground pepper to taste

2 tablespoons grated parmesan cheese

Directions:

1. Preheat oven to 400 degrees.
2. Arrange cubed bread on a baking sheet and cook for 8 minutes.
3. Cook the turkey in a medium-sized skillet over medium heat.
4. Combine milk, cheese, egg and egg substitute, onion, mushrooms, paprika, pepper and parmesan cheese in a large bowl. Add in sausage and bread cubes and mix well.
5. Pour mixture into 13x9 inch baking pan. Cover with foil and place in the refrigerator overnight or 8 hours.
6. To cook the frittata, remove foil and cook at 350 degrees for 50 minutes.

Lunch

Wheat Tuna Pitas

Ingredients

1½ cups shredded romaine lettuce

¾ cup diced tomatoes

½ cup finely chopped green bell peppers

½ cup shredded carrots

½ cup finely chopped broccoli

¼ cup finely chopped onion

2 cans (6 ounces each) low-salt white tuna packed in water, drained

½ cup low-fat ranch dressing

3 whole-wheat pita pockets, cut in half

Directions:

1. Combine lettuce, tomatoes, peppers, carrots, broccoli and onion in a bowl.
2. In a separate bowl, mix together the tuna and ranch dressing.
3. Add tuna to lettuce mixture and mix well.
4. Fill the pita pockets with the tuna mixture and serve.

Rice and Bean Salad

Ingredients

1½ cups uncooked brown rice

3 cups water

½ cup chopped fresh parsley

½ cup chopped shallots or spring onions (approximately 2 shallots or several spring onions)

15-ounce can unsalted garbanzo beans, rinsed and drained

15-ounce can unsalted dark kidney beans, rinsed and drained

¼ cup olive oil

$\frac{1}{3}$ to $\frac{1}{2}$ cup rice vinegar or as desired

Directions:

1. Cook rice in medium size pot for about 50 minutes or until done.
2. Allow rice to cool before adding in remaining ingredients.
3. Place salad in a bowl, cover and refrigerate for 2 hours.
4. Serve cold.

Spicy Chicken Salad Wraps

Ingredients

3-4 ounces of chicken breasts

2 whole chipotle peppers

$\frac{1}{4}$ cup white wine vinegar

$\frac{1}{4}$ cup low-calorie mayonnaise

2 stalks celery, diced

2 carrots, julienne style

1 small yellow onion, diced (about $\frac{1}{2}$ cup)

$\frac{1}{2}$ cup thinly sliced radish or other root vegetable

4 ounces spinach, cut into strips

2 whole-grain tortillas (12-inch diameter)

Directions:

1. Bake or grill chicken breasts. Allow to cool and then cut into cubes and set aside.
2. Place peppers, vinegar and mayonnaise in a blender and puree.
3. Place remaining ingredients (except tortillas and spinach) in a bowl and mix well.
4. Add in the chicken and puree and mix again.
5. Place spinach on each tortilla. Scoop mixture onto tortilla, wrap and eat.

Chicken and Orange Wrap

Ingredients

    8 oz chicken breast (one large breast)

    ½ cup celery, diced

    ⅔ cup canned mandarin oranges, drained

    ¼ cup onion, minced

    2 tablespoons mayonnaise

    1 teaspoon soy sauce

    ¼ teaspoon garlic powder

    ¼ teaspoon black pepper

    1 large whole wheat tortilla

    4 large lettuce leaves, washed and patted dry

Directions:

1. Bake or grill chicken breasts. Allow to cool and then cut into cubes and set aside.
2. In a medium bowl, mix chicken celery, oranges and onions.
3. Add in mayonnaise, soy sauce, garlic and pepper. Mix again until chicken is coated.
4. Cut the tortilla into 4 equal-sized triangles.
5. Put a lettuce leaf on each tortilla triangle and scoop chicken mixture onto lettuce. Fold tortilla in half (corner to corner) and serve.

Tuna Melt

Ingredients

    6 ounces white tuna packed in water, drained

    ⅓ cup chopped celery

    ¼ cup chopped onion

    ¼ cup low fat Russian or Thousand Island salad dressing

    2 whole-wheat English muffins, split

    3 ounces reduced-fat Cheddar cheese, grated

Directions:

1. Set conventional oven to broil.
2. In a bowl, combine tuna, celery, onion and salad dressing.
3. Toast muffin halves.
4. Add a scoop of tuna mixture to each muffin half. Place in oven and broil for 3 minutes.
5. Remove from oven and sprinkle cheese over the top. Return to oven for one minute, or until cheese is melted.

Caprese Salad

Ingredients

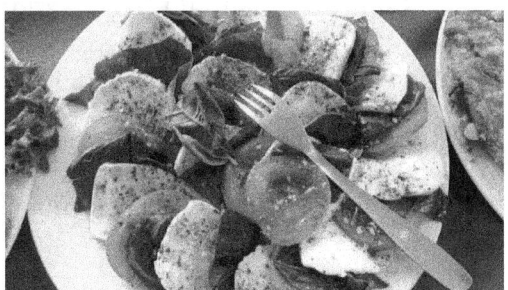

2 pounds fresh tomatoes, sliced ¼ inch thick

12-16 fresh basil leaves

3 ounces fresh mozzarella, diced

1 tablespoon balsamic vinegar

1 tablespoon extra-virgin olive oil

Fresh ground black pepper (optional)

Directions:

1. Arrange tomatoes evenly between four plates.
2. Place basil leaves between tomato slices.
3. Spread mozzarella over the top of the tomatoes.
4. In a small bowl, mix vinegar and oil.
5. Drizzle the oil mixture over the tomatoes.
6. Top with black pepper if desired.

Orange and Rice Salad

Ingredients

2 cups cooked brown rice, cooled

½ cup celery, washed and diced

¾ cup raisins or other dried fruit

¼ cup chopped nuts

2 tablespoons canola oil

1 tablespoon orange juice or vinegar

¼ cup parsley, chopped or 1 teaspoon dried parsley

3 green onions, washed and thinly sliced

1 can (11 ounces) mandarin oranges with juice

Pepper to taste

Directions:
1. Cook rice the night before and place in refrigerator.
2. Mix all ingredients into a bowl and place back in the refrigerator to chill for an hour.
3. Serve cold.

Chicken Salad

Ingredients

3¼ cups skinless chicken breast, cooked and cubed

¼ cup celery, chopped

1 tablespoon lemon juice

½ teaspoon onion powder

3 tablespoons mayonnaise, low-fat

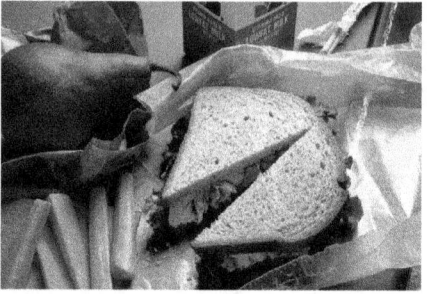

Directions:
1. Mix ingredients in a bowl. Leave in refrigerator overnight to allow flavors to blend.
2. Spread mixture on a whole wheat tortilla for a healthy wrap or use on wheat bread for a sandwich filler.

Dinner

Vegetarian Spaghetti

Ingredients

2 tablespoons olive oil

2 small onions, chopped

3 cloves garlic, chopped

1¼ cups zucchini, sliced

1 tablespoon oregano, dried

1 tablespoon basil, dried

1 8-ounce can tomato sauce

1 6-ounce can low-sodium tomato paste

2 medium tomatoes, chopped

1 cup water

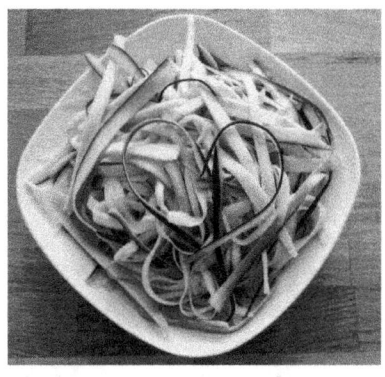

Directions:
1. Sauté onions and garlic in a stock pot.
2. Add remaining ingredients and simmer for 45 minutes.
3. Serve over whole wheat pasta.

Chicken and Rice

Ingredients

1 cup onions, chopped

¾ cup green peppers

2 teaspoons vegetable oil

1 8-ounce can tomato sauce

1 teaspoon parsley, chopped

½ teaspoon black pepper

1¼ teaspoons garlic, minced

5 cups cooked brown rice (cooked in unsalted water)

3½ cups chicken breasts, skinned and cooked, chopped

Directions:
1. Sauté onions and peppers in vegetable oil over medium heat for five minutes.
2. Add in tomato sauce, parsley pepper and garlic and heat for another 5 minutes.
3. Stir in chicken and rice. Heat for another 5 minutes and serve.

Turkey Meatloaf

Ingredients

1 pound lean ground turkey

½ cup regular oats, dry

1 large egg, whole

1 tablespoon onion, dehydrated flakes

¼ cup low-sodium ketchup

Directions:

1. Mix all ingredients in a bowl.
2. Spray a loaf pan with a low-fat cooking spray. Place mixture in pan and bake for 25 minutes at 350 degrees.

Baked Cod with Herb Crust

Ingredients

¾ cup herb-flavored stuffing

4 cod fillets, each 4 ounces

¼ cup honey

Directions:

1. Brush cod fillets with honey.
2. Place stuffing into a sealed bag and crush with a rolling pin until crumbly.
3. Place fillets, one at a time, into the bag and shake well to coat.
4. Place fillets on cooking sheet sprayed with low-fat cooking spray.
5. Bake in oven at 375 degrees for approximately 10 minutes.

Chicken and Broccoli

Ingredients

$\frac{1}{3}$ cup orange juice

1 tablespoon low-sodium soy sauce

1 tablespoon Schezuan sauce

2 teaspoons cornstarch

1 tablespoon canola oil

1 pound boneless chicken breast, cut into 1-inch cubes

2 cups of frozen broccoli florets

1 6-ounce package of frozen snow peas

2 cups shredded cabbage

2 cups of cooked brown rice

Directions:

1. Combine orange juice, soy sauce, Schezuan sauce and cornstarch in a small bowl and set aside for later.
2. Add canola oil to a wok and cook chicken for 5 minutes or until done.
3. Add vegetables and orange juice mixture to wok and cook for an additional 5 minutes.
4. Serve over brown rice.

Beef Kabobs

Ingredients

1½ pounds beef shoulder center steaks, cut 1-inch thick

Marinade:

2 tablespoons fresh lime juice

2 tablespoons olive oil

2 large cloves garlic, minced

1 medium jalapeno pepper, minced

½ teaspoon ground cumin

Pineapple Salsa:

½ medium pineapple, peeled, cored, cut into 1½-inch chunks (about 3 cups)

1 medium red onion, cut into 12 wedges

1 large red or green bell pepper, cut into 1½-inch pieces

2 teaspoons freshly grated lime peel

Directions:

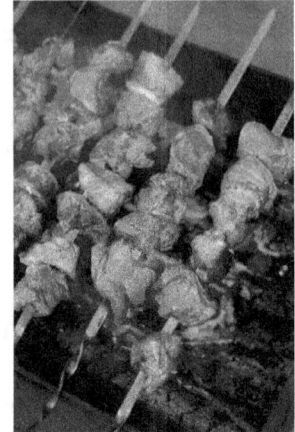

1. Mix marinade ingredients in a small bowl. Set aside 2 tablespoons to use for salsa.
2. Add meat to marinade and mix well to coat meat.
3. Place in refrigerator and allow to rest for up to 2 hours.
4. Remove meat from marinade and place on six skewers. Dispose of marinade.
5. Grill skewers for 7 to 9 minutes until meat is medium.
6. Place pineapple salsa ingredients on separate skewers by alternating layers of pineapple, onion, and bell pepper.
7. Grill fruit and vegetable skewers for 10 minutes or until veggies are soft.
8. Remove fruit and vegetables from skewers and chop to make salsa.
9. Add lime peel and marinade that was set aside.
10. Serve salsa with the skewered meat.

Shepherd's Pie

Ingredients

2 large baking potatoes, peeled and diced

½ cup low-fat milk

1 pound lean ground beef

1 medium onion, chopped

1 clove garlic, minced

2 tablespoons flour

4 cups frozen mixed vegetables

¾ cup reduced sodium beef broth

½ cup shredded cheddar cheese

ground pepper to taste

Directions:
1. Boil potatoes about 15 minutes or until soft.
2. Mash potatoes and add milk. Mix well and set aside.
3. Cook meat, onion and garlic in a skillet until meat is brown.
4. Add in flour and stir well. Pour in broth and add vegetables.
5. Continuously stir for 5 minutes over medium heat.
6. Pour vegetable mixture into an 8x8 inch pan.
7. Spread potatoes over the top.
8. Sprinkle cheese over the top of the potatoes.
9. Bake at 375 degrees for 25 minutes.

Lean Cheeseburgers

Ingredients
1 pound ground beef (95% lean)

2 tablespoons quick-cooking oats

½ teaspoon steak seasoning blend

4 seeded or whole wheat hamburger buns, split

4 slices low-fat cheese

Directions:
1. Combine beef, oats and seasoning blend in a bowl.
2. Form mixture into patties and cook on a grill until desired doneness.
3. Top with cheese, lettuce and tomatoes.

Desserts

Apples and Cream Milkshake

Ingredients
2 cups vanilla low-fat ice cream

1 cup unsweetened applesauce

¼ teaspoon ground cinnamon or apple pie spice

1 cup fat-free skim milk

Directions:

Mix all ingredients in a blender and blend until smooth.

Honey Sweetened Apples and Yogurt

Ingredients

    1 pint fresh strawberries

    4 teaspoons honey

    3 cups plain low-fat yogurt

    4 Tablespoons toasted sliced almonds

Directions:

1. Divide yogurt into four dishes.
2. Top with strawberries and drizzle with honey.
3. Sprinkle almonds on top and serve.

Berrysicles

Ingredients

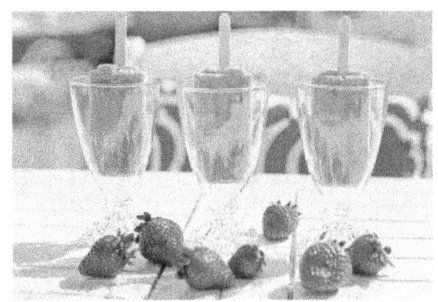

¾ cup blueberries

¾ cup blackberries

¾ cup strawberries

1 cup non-fat or low-fat plain yogurt

1¼ cup non-fat or low-fat milk

Directions:

1. Blend ingredients in a blender until smooth.
2. Pour mixture into popsicle molds until half full.
3. Freeze mixture for 30 minutes.
4. Remove from freezer, place popsicle sticks in the mixture and fill the molds to the top.
5. Place back in freezer for an additional hour or until frozen.

Brown Rice Pudding

Ingredients

3 cups 1% low-fat milk

1 cup brown rice

¼ cup sugar

1 teaspoon vanilla

¼ teaspoon almond extract

cinnamon to taste

¼ cup toasted almonds (optional)

Directions:

1. Bring milk and rice to a boil in medium saucepan.
2. Reduce heat and allow to simmer covered for 30 minutes.
3. Remove from heat and stir in sugar, vanilla, almond extract and cinnamon.
4. Top with almonds, if desired.

Peach Crisp

Ingredients

8 ripe peaches, peeled, pitted and sliced

½ teaspoon lemon juice

$1/3$ teaspoon ground cinnamon

¼ teaspoon ground nutmeg

½ cup whole-wheat flour

¼ cup packed dark brown sugar

2 tablespoons trans-free margarine, cut into thin slices

¼ cup quick-cooking oats

Directions:

1. Place sliced peaches in coated 9-inch pie pan.
2. Sprinkle lemon juice, cinnamon and nutmeg over peaches.
3. Mix flour, sugar, butter and oats in a small bowl.
4. Spread dry mixture over the peaches.
5. Bake at 375 degrees for 30 minutes.

Low-fat Cheesecake

Ingredients

2 tablespoons cold water

1 envelope unflavored gelatin

2 tablespoons lemon juice

½ cup skim milk, heated almost to boiling

1 tablespoon Egg substitute

¼ cup sugar

1 teaspoon vanilla

2 cups low-fat cottage cheese

Directions:

1. Place water, gelatin and lemon juice in a blender. Process for 2 minutes or until gelatin is thoroughly mixed.

2. Add milk and process again until gelatin is completely dissolved.
3. Add egg substitute, sugar, vanilla and cottage cheese. Process on a high speed until mixture is smooth.
4. Pour mixture into a 9-inch pie plate and place in refrigerator.
5. Allow to chill for 3 hours before serving.

Fruit Cream Dessert

Ingredients

4 ounces fat-free cream cheese, softened

½ cup plain fat-free yogurt

½ teaspoon vanilla

1 can (11 ounces) mandarin oranges, drained

1 can (8¼ ounces) water-packed sliced peaches, drained

1 can (8 ounces) water-packed pineapple chunks, drained

4 tablespoons shredded coconut, toasted

Directions:

1. Blend cream cheese, yogurt and vanilla in a bowl with a mixer on high speed.
2. In a separate bowl, mix fruit together. Gently fold in cream mixture.
3. Place in refrigerator for 2 hours before serving. Top with coconut.

Conclusion

Thank you again for purchasing this book!

I hope you have now gained valuable knowledge on your quest to better your health. The DASH Diet lifestyle change could possibly be the best thing you ever do for yourself.

If you enjoyed this book, please take the time to share your thoughts and post a review on Amazon. I would greatly appreciate it!

Thank you and good luck!

PS: You may also be interested in my other book:

The Sugar Detox Solution: A Proven Strategy for Weight Loss, Improving Your Health and Feeling Great by Defeating Your Sugar Cravings and Addiction

It's a great resource in my Healthy Life Series that I created to help you on your way to better health.

Get it on Amazon today!

Index of Recipes

www.ingramcontent.com/pod-product-compliance
Lightning Source LLC
Chambersburg PA
CBHW070228290526
45789CB00004B/1538